Renal Di

MW01231856

Newly Diagnosed

What to Expect, What to Eat, How to Thrive

By

Kate J. Ramos

Respective authors own all copyrights not held by the publisher.

The information herein is offered for informational purposes solely and is universal as so. The presentation of the information is without contract or any type of guarantee assurance.

The trademarks that are used are without any consent, and the publication of the trademark is without permission or backing by the trademark owner. All trademarks and brands within this book are for clarifying purposes only and are the owned by the owners themselves, not affiliated with this document.

Author: Kate J. Ramos

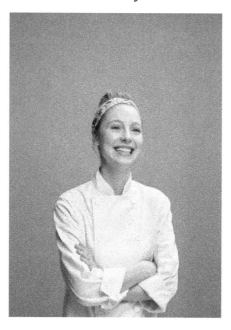

Kate J. Ramos is a registered nutritionist and dietician who uses a whole natural and food-based approach to help clients reclaim their health and improve quality of life. She has completed her dietetics teaching program at top universities in the country after achieving the clinical nutrition title. Kate J. Ramos has extensive experience working with the chronic kidney disease population. Her first introduction to renal nutrition began when she worked as a dietician in a hemodialysis facility. In this role, she was surprised to learn that most of her patients had never met a dietician before starting dialysis. It was this discovery that inspired Kate J. Ramos to start her own private practice specializing in nutritional therapy for CKD patients on pre-dialysis. Kate J. Ramos is passionate about enabling her patients to implement realistic and sustainable changes aimed at slowing the progression of their kidney disease. She continues to work with "dialysis" patients helping them to optimize their health and reduce the risk of further complications. At the same time, she was able to create a series of 7 precious works from the complete series "The Renal Diet Paradox" and they are all available... So, what are you waiting for? Cheers!

Table of Contents

Introduction

Renal diet is often called as diet for kidney or dialysis. Blood waste is produced from food and drinks that are consumed. To cut back on the volume of waste in their tissue, individuals with kidney disease must stick to a renal diet. It may also improve kidney efficiency and postpone total kidney failure after a renal diet.

One that is deficient in sodium, phosphorus and protein is a renal diet. A renal diet emphasizes the value of eating high-quality protein and reducing fluids. Restricted potassium and calcium can also be required for certain renal diets. Each person is different, so a dietician can collaborate with each patient to create a renal diet customized to their needs. For kidney health, eating correctly is essential. In specific, persons with kidney disease need to control their consumption of phosphorus, potassium, and sodium.

It's important that you monitor what you eat and drink if you do have chronic kidney disease (CKD). That's because, your kidneys do not extract waste material from your body the way it should. You will remain healthy for longer with a kidney-friendly diet.

As a standard renal diet, there is no such thing. There is no better diet than a standard renal diet. Dietary adjustments, especially restrictions, are enforced only when they are specifically required and personalized according to the age, food preferences and development of the infant. Changes to the consumption of calories, protein, fat, phosphorus, sodium, calcium, potassium and fluid may be needed. To better satisfy energy needs and to promote adherence, restrictions are maintained as liberal as possible. The restriction can be strengthened or strengthened based on the response to the specific parameter. In addition to improvements in the child's nutritional condition, age, growth, anthropometrics, food habits, residual renal activity, biochemistry, renal replacement therapy, drugs, and psychosocial status, the diet treatment strategy needs regular supervision and adjustments. Your health is influenced by what you consume and drink. It will help regulate your blood pressure and keep at a healthier weight and consume a nutritious diet low in fat and salt. You will better regulate your blood pressure if you have diabetes by consciously deciding what you consume and drink. It can help keep kidney condition from getting worse by managing diabetes and high blood pressure.

Why Renal diet is a Kidney-Friendly Diet?

The kidneys' key function is to get rid of the body's waste and excess fluid by your urine. Also, they:

- Control minerals, such as salt and potassium, in your body
- Balance the fluids in the body
- Make hormones that influence the way other organs operate.

A kidney-friendly diet is a way to eat that helps to protect the kidneys against more damage. Some minerals and fluids such as electrolytes do not build up in the body; you will have to avoid certain foods and fluids. You'll have to make sure that you get the correct amount of protein, vitamins, calories, and minerals. A kidney-friendly diet will also actually shield your kidneys from more injury. To keep the minerals in certain items from piling up in your body, a kidney-friendly diet restricts those things. It can even help improve kidney function and delay total kidney disease development by following a kidney diet. This diet aims to maintain the electrolyte, mineral, and fluid levels in your body healthy while you have or are on dialysis with CKD. To reduce the accumulation of waste material in the body, people on dialysis require this diet.

There could be little if any restrictions on what you should consume if you're in the initial CKD stages. Yet you will have to be more cautious of what you bring into your bloodstream when your condition gets worse.

For most people with severe kidney disease, a kidney-friendly diet that reduces blood waste is important to follow. The renal diet is the best diet to adopt for such circumstances. It helps to improve the function of the kidney while restricting further damage. Limit the amount of sodium to less than 2,000 mg daily. Therefore, the renal diet is ideal for CKD, i-e chronic kidney disease and other health problems such as diabetes.

The renal guideline:

The guidelines for dieting should begin with a clear description of the nutrient's function in the body, the reason for diet change, the expected effects to be obtained (e.g., normal blood pressure, clear weight gain), and what occurs if the infant consumes too much or too little of the nutrient.

Sodium: Sodium is a mineral (sodium chloride) present in salt and is commonly used in food preparation. Salt is among the most often used seasonings, although it requires time to get used to limiting the salt in the diet. Salt/sodium elimination, though, is an effective aid in managing kidney disease. In many foods, this mineral is present naturally. The most popular one is table salt.

Your blood pressure is affected by sodium. It also helps to balance the level of water in the body. Healthy kidneys hold amounts of sodium in place. Although if you have CKD, the body accumulates additional sodium and fluids. This can cause several heart and lung issues, such as elevated blood pressure, swollen ankles, fluid buildup, and shortness of breath. In your regular diet, you can settle for fewer than 2 grams of sodium.

Why should sodium consumption be controlled by kidney patients?

For individuals with kidney disease, too much salt may be dangerous since their kidneys cannot properly remove extra fluid and sodium from the body. As fluid and sodium build up in the bloodstream and tissues, they can cause:

- Elevated thirst levels•
- Edema: swelling of the thighs, hands, and face
- elevated Blood pressure

To cut the salt in your diet, follow these basic steps:

Always interpret labeling on food items. Limit foods with more than 300 mg per serving of sodium (or 600mg for a complete frozen dinner). For the first 4 to 5 foods on the product list, prevent people that contain salt.

- It always lists the sodium content
- Pay careful attention to sizes for serving.
- Use fresh meat rather than packages meat.
- Choose fresh fruit and vegetables or canned and frozen products with no-salt-added.
- Avoid the refined food items.
- Compare labels and choose the lowest-sodium products.

- Using spices that do not have "salt" in their description (prefer garlic powder instead of garlic salt.)
- Limit the average amount of sodium to 400 mg per meal and 150 mg per snack.
- Do not use salt when you are cooking food.
- Try to avoid salt on food while eating.
- Do not consume ham, pork, sausage, hot dogs, beef for lunch, nuggets or chicken tenders, or regular canned soup. Eat only soups that have logos that decrease the sodium level-and use only one cup-not the entire can.
- Choose the canned vegetables with the label "no added salt."
- Do not include salts such as garlic salt, onion salt or 'seasoned' salt that are flavored. Limit kosher or sea salt as well.
- For your favorite snacks, such as peanut butter or box mixes, make sure to check for lower salt or "no salt added" options.
- Do not buy the refrigerated or frozen meats that are processed or pre-seasoned/flavored in a solution.

Chicken breasts, burgers, pork chops, pork tenderloin, steaks are typically those products.

- Remove table salt from your diet and high-sodium seasonings like sea salt, soy sauce and garlic salt etc.

Potassium:

Potassium is a common mineral present in the food products that we consume and is naturally found in a human body. In keeping the pulse normal and the muscles functioning properly, potassium plays a part. For the preservation of fluid and electrolyte equilibrium in the bloodstream, potassium is also required. The kidneys help you keep the body's proper potassium level and remove unnecessary levels into the urine. Potassium is an element that is involved in how muscles act. Potassium builds up in the blood when the kidneys don't function properly. This will cause changes in the heartbeats, possibly eventually lead to a heart attack. Potassium is primarily present in fruits and vegetables, plus milk and beef. You would need to stop some of them and limit the number of others. It is a mineral present in most of the foods we consume and is required in the diet because it helps maintain the nervous system balanced through muscle activity. It also helps regulate the body's volume of water. In the blood, the volume of potassium is regulated by the kidneys. Potassium levels can build up to elevated levels in the blood for individuals with kidney disease. This is called hyperkalemia, and for the heart, it may be dangerous. So, an individual must reduce the consumption of potassium.

This element helps the muscles and nerves to work properly. Yet, the body can't filter all the excess potassium while you have CKD. It can result in severe cardiac attacks when you get so much of it in the blood.

Why do patients with kidneys issues have to control their intake of potassium?

Patients with kidney diseases will no longer expel surplus potassium as the kidneys collapse, so potassium levels build up in the body. High blood potassium is recognized as hyperkalemia, which may induce:

- Muscle weakness
- Slow pulse
- An irregular heart beat

- Death
- Heart attacks

How the patients can monitor potassium intake?

- A patient must control the potassium volume that reaches the body as the kidneys no longer control potassium.
- Tips to help maintain potassium levels in your blood safe by making sure:
- Speak about creating a meal schedule with a kidney dietitian.
- Restrict foods rich in potassium.
- Limit up to 8 oz a day of milk and dairy goods.
- Pick fruits and vegetables that are fresh.
- Stop sodium substitutes & potassium seasonings.
- Read labeling & prevent potassium chloride on packaged foods.
- To the serving size, pay careful attention.
- Must keep a diet journal.

Fruits and vegetables like bananas, rice, avocados, tomatoes, oranges, cooked broccoli, melons, raw carrots and greens (except kale) contain a large amount of

Potassium. These foods will influence your blood potassium levels. The doctor will let you know if you really need to restrict your dietary usage of this mineral. If so, they can suggest that you try foods with low Potassium, such as:

- Cranberries and cranberry juice
- Apples and apple juice
- Plums
- Peaches
- Pineapples
- Cabbage
- Beans (wax or green)
- Tomatoes, tomato juice and tomato sauce
- Pumpkin
- Celery
- Melons such as honeydew and cantaloupe (watermelon is okay)
- Bananas
- Prune juice
- Winter squash
- Dried beans of all kinds

- Cooked greens, collards, spinach, swiss chard and kale
- Cucumber
- Strawberries, raspberries and blueberries
- Boiled Cauliflower
- Asparagus
- Orange juice and oranges
- Grape juice

Some foods to avoid include bran cereals, granola, molasses, "salt substitute," or "lite" salt. To encourage yourself to consume sweet potatoes and potatoes in Limited quantities, they require special handling. Peel them, break them into tiny slices or squares, then soak them in a huge volume of water for many hours. Pour off the soaking water as you are about to prepare them and use a good water volume in the pan. Before you cook them to eat, drain the water. You may need to make more improvements to your diet when the CKD (chronic kidney disease) becomes worse. This may mean cutting back on high-protein foods, especially animal protein. This involves items such as beef, fish, and dairy. You may need additional iron as well. Speak to your doctor regarding which foods you should consume high in iron while you have CKD.

Phosphorus:

Phosphorus is an element important in the development and maintenance of bones. Phosphorus frequently helps grow organs and connective tissues and helps in the movement of muscles. As phosphorus-containing food is eaten and digested, phosphorus is ingested sufficiently by the small intestines to be deposited in the bones.

Phosphorus is yet another mineral that will build up in your blood when your kidneys don't function correctly. Calcium may be extracted from your bones as something occurs and may settle in your blood vessels or the skin. The bone disorder will become a concern, causing you to get a fracture in the bone more likely. It is a nutrient that we get by consuming certain foods as well. This element also helps build strong bones and teeth. It also tends to turn food into energy and helps in metabolism. Normally, kidneys expel excess phosphorus into the urine; nevertheless, kidney dysfunction may keep the body from getting rid of the accumulation that causes bone and heart issues.

Why should kidney patients monitor Phosphorus intake?

Normal functioning kidneys can extract excess phosphorus from the blood. The kidneys no more expel surplus phosphorus while kidney activity is affected. High levels of phosphorus can pull calcium from the bones, making them fragile. This often results in harmful concentrations of calcium in the blood vessels, skin, lungs and heart.

How can the patients monitor the Phosphorus intake?

In certain foods, phosphorus can be present. Therefore, to better control phosphorus amounts, patients with impaired kidney function may consult with a renal dietician. Tips for managing and retain phosphorus at healthy levels are:

- Keep in mind what foods have less phosphorus.
- Pay careful attention to the size of servings
- Eat smaller amounts of food and snacks that are rich in protein.

- Consume fresh veggies and fruits.
- Ask your doctor to utilize phosphate binders when eating.
- Avoid processed food with additional phosphorus. On ingredient labels, check the phosphorus level or the terms with "PHOS."
- Must keep a diet log

The main phosphorus source in the diet is dairy products, so restrict milk to 1 cup per day. Just one glass or 1 ounce a day if you use cheese or yogurt instead of liquid milk!

Phosphorus is also present in certain vegetables. Limit the dried beans, greens, mushrooms, broccoli and Brussels sprouts to 1 cup each week. There is a need to restrict these cereals to 1 serving a week: cereals, wheat, oatmeal, bran and granola. White bread is healthier than bread or crackers produced from whole grains.

Soft beverages contain phosphorus, so only clear drinks are available. Do not consume some Mountain Dew, cola, root beer, Dr. Pepper (any kind). Hawaiian Punch, cool iced tea, Fruit works, and Aquafina tangerine pineapple are also resisted. Alcohol has phosphorus too, avoid all forms.

Protein

For safe kidneys, protein isn't a concern. Protein is usually absorbed, and excess waste products are produced, purified by the kidney nephrons. Then, the waste transforms into the urine with the aid of additional renal proteins. On the other side, damaged kidneys fail to eliminate protein waste, and it accrues in the blood.

For Chronic Kidney Disorder patients, adequate protein intake is tricky since the volume changes with each disease level. Protein is necessary to maintain tissues and other bodily roles, but according to the nephrologist or kidney dietician, it is vital to consume the prescribed amount for the stage of the disease.

Fluids

The Fluid control is important for patients in the later stages of Chronic Kidney Disease because fluid consumption may cause fluid buildup in the body which could become dangerous. People on dialysis usually have lower urine output, so increased number fluid in the body can put unusual pressure on the person's lungs and heart.

The patient's fluid count is calculated on an individual basis, depending upon the output of urine and setting of dialysis. It is essential to follow the nutritionist's or nephrologist's fluid intake instructions.

- To control the fluid intake, patients should:
- Do not drink alcohol more than the doctor suggests.
- Count all foods (popsicles, Jell-O etc.) that can melt at room temp.
- Be aware of the number of fluids used in the preparation of food

Chapter no: 1 Renal-friendly breakfast recipes

You can enjoy delicious home-made quick breakfast recipes while following Renal diet plan. Some of them are listed below. So, what are you waiting for? Go grab the ingredient and make these quick kidney friendly recipes and fulfill your appetite.

1.1 No Fuss Microwave Egg White French Toast

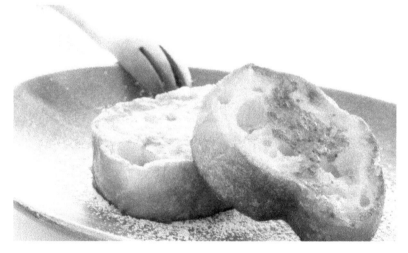

Portion: 1

Serving size: 1

Diet types include CKD non-dialysis, Diabetes, Lower protein and Dialysis

Total time: 10min

Ingredients:

- 1/2 cup of egg whites
- 1 slice of a bread
- 2 tablespoons of sugar-free syrup
- 1 teaspoon of softened unsalted butter

Preparation:

1. Around English muffin or bread, spread some butter. Chopped into cubes.

2. In a microwave-safe dish, put the cubes of buttered bread.

3. To cover, spill the egg whites over the bread.

4. Sprinkle the syrup over the top

5. Microwave it for 1 minute; press the white egg's sides to the edges to allow the uncooked egg out.

6. Microwave for an additional minute or until the egg is set.

Some Helpful hints:

1 Serve it warm as French toast or cool and serve as bread pudding.

2 Egg whites have minimum phosphorus or fat and high-quality protein.

3 Substitute   beaten 1/2-cup of egg   white or 2 whole eggs if necessary. The shift raises nutrients to 288 calories, 434 mg of cholesterol, 15 g of fat, 226 mg of phosphorus and decreases sodium to 353 mg.

4 Substitute lite or sugar-free syrup with cinnamon sugar or real maple syrup if needed.

5 This recipe goes best for half of an English muffin instead of a bread slice.

1.2 Yummy Omelet in just 40-seconds

Eggs are a best protein source and a quick meal when you have limited time.

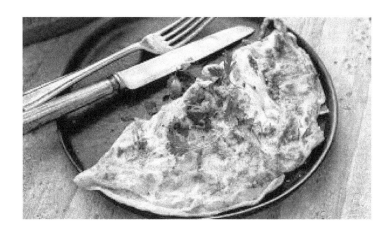

Portion: 1

Serving size: 2

Total time: 10min

Ingredients:

Based on 1 serving per recipe.

- 2tablespoons of water
- eggs
- 1/2 cup of filling (meat, vegetables and seafood)
- 1tablespoon of unsalted butter

Preparation:

1. Whip the eggs and water together until mixed.

2. Heat butter in a 10-inch fry pan or omelet pan until just hot enough for a drop of water to sizzle.

3. Pour the egg mixture onto it. The mixture should be set on the edges instantly. Move cooked portions cautiously at the edges into the middle using an upright pancake turner so that uncooked portions will touch the hot pan surface. Tilt the pan and transfer as needed.

4. Continue until the egg is set and does not flow. If required, fill the omelet with half a cup of vegetables, beef, or seafood stuffing. If you are right-handed, place the filling on the left side, and if you're left-handed, on the right side.

5. Fold the omelet in half using the pancake turner. Invert the omelet's bottom side facing up onto a tray.

1.3 **1.3** Renal friendly Loaded Veggie Eggs

It is a versatile renal friendly breakfast recipe that increases your low potassium intake of vegetables.

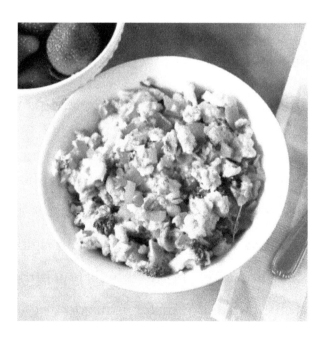

Serving size: 2 persons

Portion: 1/2 recipe

Total time: 10min

Ingredients:

- 1 cup of cauliflower
- 4 whole eggs
- Spring onion and fresh parsley for garnish
- 1 garlic clove which must be minced
- 1/4 tsp of black pepper
- 1/4 cup of chopped onion
- cups of fresh spinach
- 1 tbsp of oil of your choice (avocado oil or coconut out is better for high heat)
- 1/4 c of bell pepper which must be chopped
- *optional tomatoes on the side if there is no potassium restriction

Preparation:

1 beat the eggs and pepper until soft and fluffy and then set aside
2 Heat the oil in a broad skillet over medium heat.

3   In the skillet, add the onions and peppers and sauté until the peppers are crispy and golden.

4   Add the garlic, stir rapidly to mix, and add the cauliflower and spinach immediately.

5   Turn the heat to medium-low, sauté the vegetables and cover for some minutes.

6   Add the eggs and whisk to combine with the vegetables.

7   Cover it with spring onions or fresh parsley when the eggs are fully fried. You can serve with a side of fresh tomatoes covered with cracked black pepper if there is no potassium limit. With these, a touch of feta or a nice sharp cheese will also be delicious.

1.4 1.4 Egg and Sausage Breakfast Sandwich

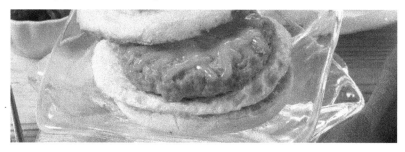

Portions: 1

Serving Size: 1 sandwich

Diet Types: Lower protein, Diabetes, CKD non-dialysis and dialysis

Total time: 15min

Ingredients

- 1 English muffin
- 1 tablespoon of natural sharp cheddar cheese which must be shredded
- 1/4 cup of low-cholesterol liquid egg substitute
- nonstick cooking spray
- A turkey sausage patty

Preparation

1. Pour the egg product into a small pan coated with nonstick cooking spray and cook over medium-low heat. Turn over the side with a spatula and cook for an extra 30 seconds until the egg is nearly cooked through

2. Toast the English muffin

3. Put the turkey sausage patty on a tray, cover with a paper towel, and cook for a minute in the microwave or the recommended time on the package.

4. Assemble the cooked eggs on the muffin and fold them to fit the muffin. Cover it with patty sausage, sharp cheddar cheese and half the leftover muffin.

Some Helpful hints:

- A fast-food sausage egg sandwich produces 800 to 1,135 mg of sodium, 30 grams of fat, 280 mg of phosphate and 255 mg of cholesterol for comparison.
- Replacing eggs with low-cholesterol egg items tends to minimize fat, cholesterol and phosphorus.
- English muffin size: 2 oz; the size of turkey patty sausage: 1 oz. Search for the lowest sodium content sausage.

1.5 1.5 Stuffed Breakfast Biscuits

Grab a biscuit with tea. These delicious biscuits, filled with eggs, cheddar cheese and bacon, are great for a weekend meal.

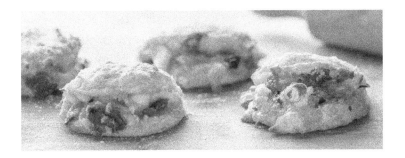

Serving size: 12

Portion: 1

Total time: 20min

Ingredients:

- 1 tablespoon of or honey or sugar
- 2 cups of flour
- ¾ cup of milk
- ½ teaspoon of baking soda
- tablespoons of softened unsalted butte
- 1 tablespoon of lemon juice

Filling includes:

- 4 eggs
- 1 cup of shredded Cheddar cheese
- oz (1¼ chopped) reduced-sodium bacon

- ¼ cup of thinly sliced scallions

Preheat the oven to 425° F.

Preparation:

To prepare the filling:

1 Slightly cook the Scrambled eggs.

2 Cook the bacon until it becomes crispy.

3 Combine all four ingredients together and set them aside.

To prepare the dough:

1 Combine all the dried ingredients in a large bowl.

2 Cut with a pastry cutter or fork in unsalted butter until smaller or pea-size.

3 In the middle of the mixture, make a well and knead in the milk and lemon juice.

4 Organize muffin tins with a liner or gently grease and flour the sides and bottom.

5 Scoop 1/4 cup of mix in the muffin tins.

6 Bake for 10-12 minutes until golden brown at 425° F.

1.6 1.6 Stuffed Poblano Pepper Recipe

With all your favorite breakfast products, these mildly spicy poblano peppers are packed to the full. Crispy Hash browns, soft scrambled eggs Speckled with sun dried scallions, tomatoes and cheese

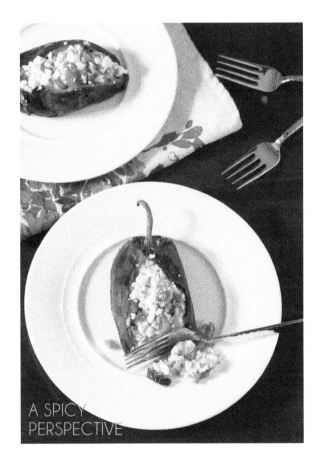

Serving size: 2

Portion: 1

Total time: 15min

Ingredients:

- Hash browns
- 2eggs
- ½ cup Shredded cheese
- Poblano peppers
- Tomatoes

Preparation:

1 Start by baking poblano peppers in the microwave until the pepper is bubbly on the outside.

2 Heat a skillet on the stovetop when the peppers are frying to prepare the hash browns. In the skillet, melt some butter and brown the hash browns till they become crispy and golden.

3 The next move is to crack the eggs and whisking them together until they are foamy. Then add the sun-dried scallions, tomatoes and quesadilla cheese

4 Over the Hash browns, pour the egg mixture and mix them. The eggs will cook fast until the eggs are undercooked but still scoop able; you can take them off the heat to stuff the peppers.

1.7 1.7 Kidney friendly egg breakfast

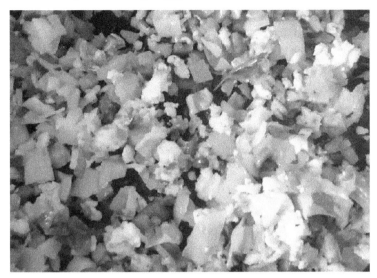

Portion: 1

Serving size: 2

Total time: 10min

Ingredients:

- Parsley
- egg whites
- Black pepper
- ¼ cup of mushrooms
- 2tbsp of small dices jalapeno
- ¼ cup of chopped cabbage

- 2tbsp of small diced bell pepper

Preparation:

1. Sautee all until fragrant; at last, add mushrooms. You always like your vegetables to have a crunch.
2. Combine the eggs with garlic and seasoning. fry on a medium-low flame
3. Sprinkle fresh parsley on the top.

Chapter 2: Renal-friendly Lunch recipes

While it may be challenging to move into a healthy lifestyle, taking tiny measures will help you step on the right path. You will typically find all the food you need at the nearest supermarket and grocery store near you. To make healthy meals, you only need to learn what foods to get. Needless to mention, it can allow you to recover and reduce the chances of further kidney issues by consuming nutritious foods, coupled with daily exercise, and will help enhance your kidney (and general) safety for years to come. So here are some delicious recipes which you can make and enjoy while following a renal diet plan.

1.8 2.1 Tortilla Beef Rollups

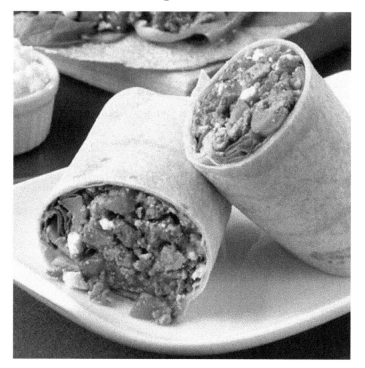

Portions: 2

Diet Types: Dialysis and Diabetes

Serving Size: 4 pieces or 1 rollup

Total time: 15min

Ingredients:

- 6" size 2 flour tortillas

- tbsp of whipped cream cheese

- 5oz cooked roast beef

- 1/4 cup of chopped red onion
- 1/4 strips of sweet bell pepper (yellow, green and red)
- slices of cucumber
- leaves of romaine lettuce
- 1 teaspoon of Mrs. Dash herb seasoning blend

Preparation:

1. Spread the cream cheese onto the tortillas.

2. To make 2 tortillas, divide the supplies in half. Layer the roast beef, pepper strips, red onion, lettuce and cucumber on each tortilla.

3. Sprinkle with the spice seasoning blend from Mrs. Dash®.

4. As a jellyroll, rollback.

Cut four pieces of each tortilla or serve whole.

Helpful hints

- Rollups stay well for up to 2 days in the refrigerator. Make it ahead and consume it as a quick lunch or high-protein snack.

- Whipped cream cheese stretches more quickly than normal cream cheese.

- To compare the sodium content, check the tortilla labels pick the lowest sodium brand.

1.9 2.2 Crunchy Chicken Wraps

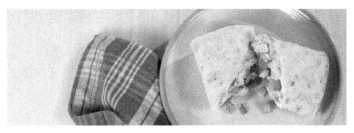

Portions: 4

Diet Types include: Diabetes, lower protein, CKD non-dialysis and Dialysis.

Serving Size: 1/2 wrap

Totaltime: 20min

Ingredients:

- A medium carrot
- A stalk celery
- 1/4 cup of mayonnaise low in fats
- oz low-sodium canned chicken
- 1/2 red bell pepper

- whole wheat tortillas, 8-inch in size or 2 whole wheat lavash
- 1/2 teaspoon of onion powder

Preparation:

1. Dice carrot, celery and bell pepper.

2. Mix the onion powder and mayonnaise in a bowl.

3. Spread two tbsp of the mixture over each flatbread or one tablespoon of the mixture over each tortilla.

4. Combine the diced vegetables in a separate bowl.

5. Place one side of each flatbread with half of the vegetables and four chicken oozes. Place 1/4th of the vegetables and 2 ounces of chicken on one side of every tortilla while using a tortilla.

6. Roll the flatbread up and diagonally cut each one in half. With a toothpick, secure each half. Secure every other tortilla with a toothpick when using a tortilla instead of lavash and cut each tortilla roll in half before actually serving.

Helpful hints:

- If low-sodium canned chicken is not available, substitute with baked pieces of chicken or fresh stewed
- Compare the products and choose the lowest sodium tortilla or lavash.

1.10 2.3 Brewery Burger

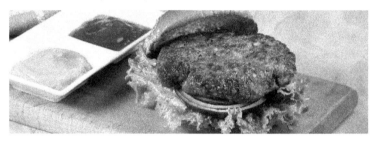

Portions: 4

Diet Types: Dialysis and Diabetes

Serving Size: 3-1/2 oz

Total time: 15min

Ingredients

- salt-free soda crackers
- tbsp of rice milk
- 1 teaspoon of salt-free herbs seasoning blend
- A large egg
- 1 pound of ground beef, must be 85% lean

Preparation

1. Crush the soda crackers and then mix them in a cup with the milk. Let the crackers stand until they are fluffy.

2. Beat and whisk the egg into the cracker mixture. Add the herb blend; combine well, breaking the crackers if required. Add the ground beef and then mix thoroughly.

3. Pat the mixture of ground beef into 4 patties of similar size.

4. Grill until cooked, over medium heat, until the core temperature is at least 160o F.

5. Serve on a bun with the desired toppings or serve with your choice's vegetable and starch.

Helpful hints

- Always cook the ground beef at a temperature of at least 160° F.
- Nutrient analysis does not include toppings, bun and side dishes.

1.11   2.4 Shrimp Quesadilla

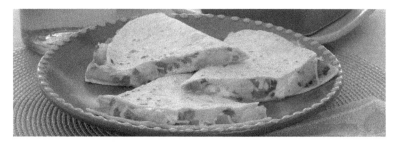

Portions: 2

Diet types include: Lower protein, Diabetes, Dialysis and CKD non-dialysis

Serving Size: 1 tortilla or 4 pieces

Total time: 15min

Ingredients

- tablespoons of jalapeno shredded cheddar cheese
- tablespoons of cilantro
- oz raw shrimp
- 1 tablespoon of lemon juice
- 1/8 teaspoon of cayenne pepper
- 1/4 teaspoon of ground cumin
- tablespoons of sour cream
- flour tortillas of burrito size
- teaspoons of salsa

Preparation

1. Devein and shell shrimp. Rinse and cut into bite-size pieces. Chop the cilantro.

2. In a zip-lock bag, combine cilantro, cumin, lemon juice, and cayenne pepper to make your marinade. Add the pieces of shrimp and set them aside to marinate for 5 minutes.

3Heat a pan over medium heat and add the marinade with the shrimp. Stir-fry the shrimp for 1 to 2 minutes until it turns orange. Remove the pan from the heat and spoon out the shrimp, leaving the marinade.

4. To marinate in the skillet, add the sour cream and stir to combine.

5. Heat the tortillas in a microwave or skillet. Spread each tortilla with two teaspoons of salsa. Top with a mixture of 1/2 shrimp and then sprinkle with 1 tablespoon of cheese.

6. Spoon 1 tablespoon of sour cream on top of the shrimp marinade mixture. Fold the tortilla in half, heat it in the baking dish, then remove it from the pan. Repeat with the

second tortilla and the shrimp, cheese and marinade remaining.

7. Cut the tortilla into 4 pieces each. When ready to serve, garnish it with cilantro and lemon wedge.

1.12   2.5 BBQ Chicken Pita Pizza

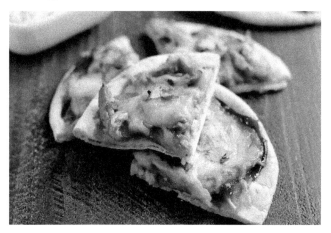

Serving Size: 1 pita pizza

Portions: 2

Diet types includes: Dialysis, CKD non-dialysis and Diabetes

Total time: 15min

Ingredients

- tablespoons of low-sodium barbecue sauce
- pita breads, 6-1/2 inches in size

- oz cooked chicken
- 1/4 cup of purple onion
- 1/8 teaspoon of garlic powder

Preparation

1 Preheat the oven at 350° F.

2 Layer the baking sheet with some cooking spray and then place 2 pitas on the sheet.

3 Spread 1-1/2 tablespoon of BBQ sauce on each pita.

4 Dice the onion and spread it over pitas.

5 Dice the chicken and layer it on the pitas.

6 Sprinkle some garlic powder and feta cheese over pitas.

7 Bake for about 11 to 13 min.

Some helpful hints:

- Eat pita pizzas immediately after baking; they will become too crispy otherwise.
- Review the nutrition labeling and purchase the feta cheese and pitas brand with the lowest sodium level.

1.13   2.6 Soft Tacos with Mexican Seasoning

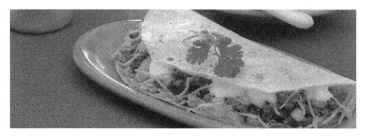

Portions: 7

Diet types include: Diabetes, CKD non-dialysis and Dialysis

Serving Size: 2 tacos

Total time: 15min

Ingredients

- cups of lettuce
- tablespoons of onion
- 1/2 cup of low-sodium tomato sauce
- 1 pound of ground beef
- tablespoons of sharp cheddar cheese, must be shredded
- 14 flour tortillas of 6-inch
- tablespoons of sour cream

Preparation

1. Make the recipe for Mexican Seasoning

2. Chop the lettuce and onion.

3. brown the ground beef and then drain it. Add the mix of spices and the tomato sauce, which is low in sodium. Heat over moderate flame and then warm up tortillas.

4. Take 1 flour tortilla and add 1/4 cup of seasoned ground beef, 1 teaspoon of cheese, 1 teaspoon of sour cream, 1 teaspoon of onion and lettuce as required to assemble soft tacos.

Helpful hints

Vegetarian ground meat or ground turkey can be used as a substitute instead of the ground beef.

1.14   2.7 Leached Mashed Potatoes with Roasted Garlic

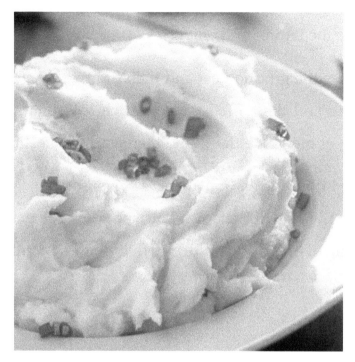

Portions: 2

Diet types include Diabetes, Gluten Free, Chronic Kidney Disease, PCOS, Nut Free, and it is low in sodium and potassium

Serving size: 4

Total time: 20min

Ingredients:

- 1 garlic
- large peeled and diced potatoes

- 1 tbsp of olive oil
- 1/4 cup of milk
- 1 tbsp of butter
- chives for garnishing
- black pepper
- parsley for garnishing

Preparation:

1. Preheat the oven to 400°F. Put the potato and fill it with cool water in a bowl, then bring it to a boil.

2. In the meantime, cut the top part of the garlic such that the cloves are revealed, and olive oil is drizzled on it. Place it in the oven and cover it in aluminum foil. Roast for thirty min, until golden brown and softened.

3. Pour the water out and add fresh water to wash the potatoes after the potatoes finally come to a simmer. Get it back to a boil and continue to cook until the potatoes are tender. Entirely drain the potatoes. Add the butter, milk, and the quantity of garlic needed. use half a head of garlic

4. Get the potatoes mashed. To taste, season with pepper. Garnish with parsley or chives.

Helpful hint:

you can leach, soak or cutup the potatoes in the water to decrease the potassium content present in the potatoes.

1.15   2.8 Chicken Broccoli Stromboli

It is mix chicken with red pepper, fresh garlic, basil, broccoli, oregano and grated mozzarella. Then wrap it up in the yummy pizza dough and the bake it to perfection.

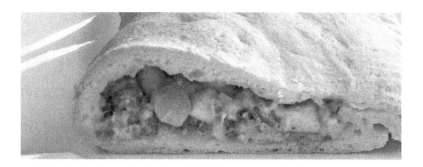

Serving size: 4

Portion: 1

Total time: 10min

Ingredients:

- cups of fresh broccoli florets
- 1-pound pizza dough
- cups of diced cooked chicken breast
- 1 tablespoon fresh garlic, chopped

- 1 cup of low-salt shredded mozzarella cheese
- 1 tablespoon of fresh chopped oregano
- tablespoons of flour
- 1 teaspoon of crushed red chili flakes
- tablespoons of olive oil

Preparation:

1. In a large bowl, mix the chicken, pepper flakes, cheese, broccoli, oregano and garlic and set aside.

2. Flour dust the tabletop and roll the dough out until you reach a rectangular form of 11" x 14".

3. Place the chicken mixture along the longest line, about 2 inches from the dough's edge.

4. Roll and pinch the ends and seam when sealed securely (a fork can be used to crimp the edges for a tight seal).

5. Using olive oil to brush the top and make three narrow slits on the dough's top.

6. Bake on the lightly oiled baking sheet tray for 8-12 minutes or until golden brown.

7. Remove, leave for 3-5 minutes to rest, then cut and serve.

1.16   2.9 Chicken Fajitas

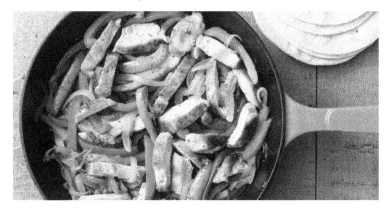

Portions: 4

Diet types include: Diabetes, CKD non-dialysis and Dialysis

Serving size: 2 fajitas

Total time: 15min

Ingredients:

- 1/4 cup of green pepper
- flour tortillas of 6" size
- tablespoons of lemon juice
- 1/4 cup of red pepper
- 1/2 cup of cilantro
- 1/2 cup of onion
- teaspoons of chili powder

- tablespoons of canola oil
- 1/4 teaspoon of black pepper
- 12 oz boneless chicken breast
- 1/2 teaspoons of cumin

Preparation:

Preheat the oven at 300° F. Roll up the tortillas in an aluminum foil and then heat in microwave oven for about 10 min.

Dice the onion, peppers and cilantro. Cut the chicken breasts into 1inch strips.

3. Place some oil over medium heat in the nonstick frying pan; add the chicken, lemon juice and seasonings. For 3 to 5 minutes, cook it.

4. In the frying pan, add the onion and peppers; cook for 3 to 5 more minutes or until the chicken is no pinker and the juice is evident. Add the cilantro to the chicken mix.

5. Divide the mixture of chicken between the tortillas and then fold the tortillas over.

Helpful hints:

For the lower protein diet lower the chicken portion to match it with your meal plan.

1.17   2.10 Chicken and Gnocchi Dumplings

Fresh gnocchi are used as the dumplings in this tasty, easy and quick chicken soup.

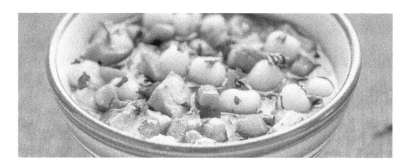

Serving size: 10

Portion: 1

Diet type includes: Diabetes and dialysis

Total time: 20min

Ingredients:

- 1 pound of gnocchi
- pounds of chicken breast
- ¼ cup of light olive oil or grape seed
- cups of low-sodium chicken stock

- 1 tablespoon low sodium Better Than Bouillon Chicken Base
- ½ cup of finely diced fresh celery
- ½ cup of finely diced fresh carrots
- ½ cup of finely diced fresh onions
- 1 teaspoon of Italian seasoning
- ¼ cup of chopped fresh parsley
- 1 teaspoon of black pepper

Preparation:

1. Put the stockpot on the stove, add the oil, and set it to heat.

2. Put the chicken in the hot oil and brown until it is golden brown on all sides

3. Add the celery, onions and carrots and cook until translucent with the chicken. Add the chicken stock and then let it cook for 20-30 minutes on high heat.

4. now, Add the chicken bouillon, Italian seasoning and black pepper, minimize the heat and then stir. Add the gnocchi and cook, stirring continuously, for 15 minutes.

5. Remove it from the stove, add the parsley and serve.

1.18   2.11 Fired Zucchini Turkey Burger

Get the grill and with these snappy, zucchini-turkey burgers, fire up the taste buds. Toss fresh poblano peppers at the grill until they're blistered, and then cover the burgers with them for some extra zing.

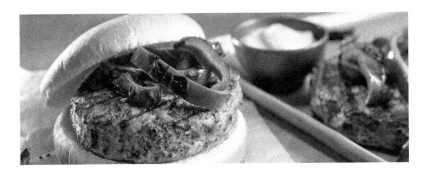

Serving size: 4

Portion: 1

Diet types include CKD non-dialysis and Diabetes

Total time: 20min

Ingredients:

- 1 cup of shredded zucchini
- 1 pound of ground turkey meat
- ½ cup of minced onion

- 1 egg
- 1 sliced, minced and seeded jalapeño pepper
- fresh seeded and sliced in half length wise poblano peppers
- 1 teaspoon of Mrs. Dash Extra Spicy Blend
- 1 teaspoon of mustard, optional

Preparation:

1. Thoroughly mix the first six ingredients. Shape meat mixture into Four patties of turkey burger.
2. Turkey burgers can be cooked on a grill or an electronic griddle.
3. When the skin becomes blistered and tender, you can grill the peppers with turkey burgers.
4. Grill turkey burgers at an internal temperature of 165 ° F or until the core is no longer pink.
5. Serve on a hamburger bun with topped patty and sliced grilled peppers, and then serve.

Chapter no 3: Renal-friendly dinner recipes

A wooden spoon, skillet and fresh ingredients are all you really need to prepare one of these simple, nutritious renal friendly dishes for your dinner. Although conventional stir-fry recipes demand higher-sodium sauces, this kidney friendly plan has low-sodium content and loaded with flavors. Bring out the skillet and start cooking and enjoy these tasty recipes for your dinner.

1.19 3.1 Vegetarian kidney friendly Shepherd's Pie

This is a short and simple recipe. Christine's tip of flipping a mashed potato filling for couscous not just saves a lot of time but helps make this tomato-based dish suitable for a renal diet.

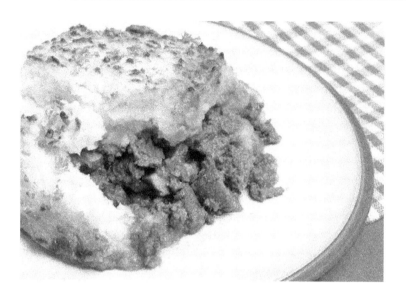

Serving size: 4

Portion: 1

Diet types include CKD non-dialysis and diabetes

Total time: 10min

Ingredients:

- 400g or 16oz can have rinsed and drained chickpeas in water
- 300g or 12oz tin of rinsed and drained lentils in water
- cups of boiled frozen vegetables
- 1 teaspoon of paprika

- 400g or 16oz can of diced tomatoes with juice drained and then discarded
- Some freshly ground black pepper
- 250g or12oz couscous 60g or 2oz hard grated cheese, grated

Preparation:

1 Put the mixed frozen vegetables and bring them to a boil in a big pan of cold water. For 5 minutes, cook them, rinse and discard the water.

2 Meanwhile, put all the other ingredients into a pan and heat through, except the cheese and couscous.

3 Add the cooked vegetables. Put it in an oven-resistant dish.

4 Following the directions on the packet, cook the couscous and sprinkle over the dish. Sprinkle the cheese over the couscous and grill before golden brown.

5 serve with some crusty bread

1.20 3.2 Jollof Rice

This is a simple edition of the popular rice dish served in so many West African parts, making an outstanding side dish to fish and meat.

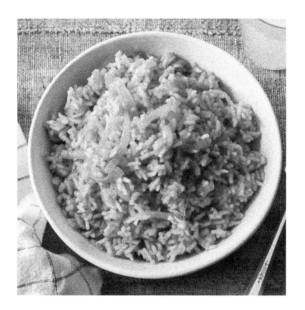

Portion: 1

Serving size: 2

Total time: 20min

Ingredients:

- 1/2 salt stock cube
- 1 medium peeled and chopped tomato
- 100g or 4oz long brown or white grain rice

- teaspoons vegetable oil
- 1 medium chopped onion (optional)
- 1 minced red chili pepper
- 1 clove of minced garlic (optional)

Preparation:

1 Bring the rice to a 5-minute boil.

2 To extract the extra starch, drain and rinse it with cold water.

3 With the stock cube, put the rice to a boil again here in 200ml/1/3 pint of water.

4 Mix the tomatoes, spicy chili peppers (onion and garlic, if necessary) and vegetable oil.

5 Cook for about 30-40 minutes or before it absorbs the water.

6 Serve with grilled white fish and a side salad mixture.

1.21   3.3 Renal friendly Low-sodium Honey-Garlic Marinade Kebabs

A quick marinade of sweet and savory kebab, perfect for a renal diet. Over the summer, grilled kebabs are a delicious dish to serve (and eat!). They are enjoyable to eat while time-consuming to put together, so more than kidney friendly. For the renal diet, these kebabs are perfect. For patients with newly diagnosed kidney disease, kebabs are one of our preferred "less meat meals" since you can still bulk up a kebab with loads of vegetables and keep the meat low. However, you can still make meat-exclusive kebabs to go with the veggie ones if you're on dialysis and looking for Even more nutrition.

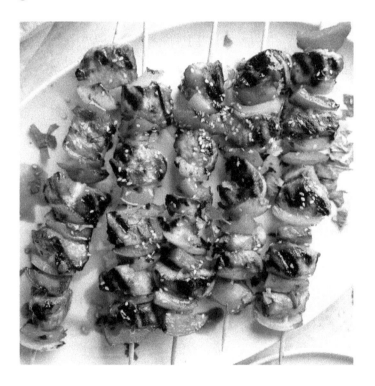

Serving size: 2

Portion: 1

Total time: 15min

Ingredients:

- crushed cloves of garlic
- 1/3 c of honey
- 1/4 c of olive oil
- 1/4 tsp of black pepper
- 1/4 c of Bragg's Liquid Amines
- This kebab marinate is best for maximum 4 medium chicken breasts, 3 peppers and 4 small onions. (max 15-20 kebabs)

Preparation:

1. In a plastic jar, combine all the ingredients.

2. For maximum 30 minutes, add prepared kebabs or meat to marinate, ideally overnight.

3. For the first 5 minutes of preparation, use the marinade to baste the kebabs.

1.22 3.4 Easy Chicken and Pasta Dinner

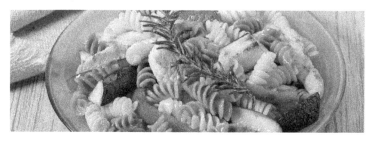

Portions: 2

Diet Types include: Diabetes, Dialysis and CKD non-dialysis

Serving size: 1 cup of pasta, 2/3 cup of vegetables and 2-1/2 oz of chicken

Total time: 20min

Ingredients:

- 1/2 cup of sliced red bell pepper
- 1 tablespoon of olive oil
- cups of cooked pasta of any shape
- tablespoons of Italian low-sodium dressing
- 1 cup sliced zucchini
- ounces of cooked chicken breast

Preparation:

1. Heat the olive oil in a nonstick skillet and sauté the peppers and zucchini until soft and crisp. Simply remove to a plate.

2. Take some Chicken, sliced into strips.

3. In different pans, heat chicken strips and cooked pasta in a microwave.

4. Toss spaghetti with Italian seasoning. Add sautéed vegetables and chicken strips at the end.

Some helpful hints:

- Do a little pre-preparation to make a fast dinner with this. To be used in this recipe and other pasta dishes, cook a big pot of pasta, rinse, and refrigerate.

- Barbeque or broil a pound of breasts or thighs of the chicken. For this recipe, as well as other chicken recipes, refrigerate and use them throughout the week.

- Adjust the chicken portion in this dish if you require a reduced protein diet.

1.23   3.5 Smothered Pork Chops and Sautéed Greens

Southern palette comfort. Crispy pan-fried pork chops, doused with sautéed onions, paprika, some seasoning, garlic and scallions and eaten with the side of sautéed collard green

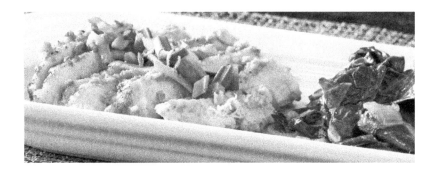

Serving size: 6 (1 serving = 1/6 sautéed greens, 1 pork chop)

Portion: 1

Total time: 20min

Ingredients:

Smothered Chops of Pork:

- 1 tablespoon of black pepper
- pork loin chops ("natural" bone-in and center cut)
- teaspoons of granulated onion powder
- 1 cup of flour
- ½ cup sliced on the bias fresh scallions
- teaspoons of paprika
- teaspoons of granulated garlic powder
- ½ cup of canola oil

- 1 ½ cups of sliced fresh onions

Sautéed Greens:

- tablespoons of olive oil
- ¼ cup finely diced onions
- 1 tablespoon of chopped fresh garlic
- 1 teaspoon of vinegar
- cups of chopped and blanched fresh collard greens
- 1 teaspoon of crushed red pepper flakes
- 1 tablespoon of unsalted butter
- 1 teaspoon of black pepper

Preparation:

Preheat the oven to 350° F.

Pork Chops:

1. Mix together the black pepper, paprika, powdered onion and garlic powder. Use half of the mixture for dressing both sides of pork chops and combine the remaining half with 1 cup of flour.

2. For later, save 2 teaspoons of the flour mixture.

3. Coat the pork chops lightly with seasoned flour.

4. Heat oil in a large oven-ready sauté tray (no rubber handles) or Dutch oven on medium flame

5. Fry the pork chops on either side for 2-4 minutes or until the desired crispness is achieved. Take it out of the pan and pour all but 2 teaspoons of oil out.

6. Cook the onions for around 4-6 minutes until translucent. Stir in 2 teaspoons of the reserved flour and stir well for around 1 minute with the onions.

7. Add the beef stock slowly and mix until it thickens.

8. Place the pork chops back in the pan and coat them with sauce. Cover or seal with foil and bake in the oven at 350° F for at least 30-45 minutes.

9. Remove from the oven and leave to rest before serving for at least 5-10 minutes.

Sautéed Greens:

1. Add the greens to a bowl of hot water for about 30 seconds to blanch the greens.

2. Strain the boiling water and transfer it quickly to a ready bowl of water and ice.

3. Let the greens cool, and strain and dry, then put aside.

4. Melt the oil and butter together in a wide saucepan over medium-high flame. Add the garlic and onions and simmer for around 4-6 minutes, until golden brown.

5. Add the red pepper, collard greens, and black pepper, then simmer on high heat for 5-8 minutes while stirring continuously.

6. remove it from the heat; apply, if you want, add vinegar and stir.

1.24   3.6 Speedy Chicken Stir-Fry

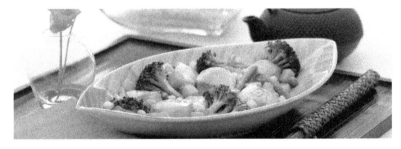

Portions: 6

Diet Types include: Lower protein, Dialysis, Diabetes and CKD-non dialysis

Serving Size: 1/2 cup of vegetables, 2 ounces of chicken and 1/2 cup of rice

Ingredients:

- cups of hot cooked rice
- tablespoons of honey
- 12 ounces of skinless and boneless chicken breast
- cups of mixed frozen vegetables
- tablespoons of pineapple juice
- 1-1/2 teaspoon of cornstarch
- tablespoons of vinegar
- 1-1/2 tablespoon of low-sodium soy sauce
- 2 tablespoons of canola oil

Preparation:

1.   Rinse the chicken and then pat it off. Cut the chicken into 1-inch parts and set aside.

2. Stir the vinegar, honey, soy sauce, pineapple juice, and cornstarch to make the sauce and set it aside.

3. In a large wok or skillet, add canola oil. (As required during cooking, add more oil.) Preheat over medium-high heat.

4. Stir-fry the frozen vegetables for about 3min or until the vegetables become crisp-tender.

5. Take the vegetables out of the skillet.

6. Add the chicken to the heavy saucepan. Stir-fry for 3-4 min or until there is no more pink chicken. Push the chicken out of the middle of the skillet. Stir the sauce and add it to the center of the skillet. Cook and mix until bubbly and thickened.

7. Placed the cooked vegetables back in the skillet. To coat, stir all the ingredients together. Cook and mix for another 1 minute or until heated.

8. Serve over rice immediately.

Some helpful hints:

Select some frozen veggie mixture of red peppers, broccoli, mushroom and bamboo or try some red peppers, green beans or water chestnuts.

1.25   3.7 Crusted-Pesto Catfish

Love the catfish, just eager for some crunch? Cook it up with mozzarella, flaky   panko   breadcrumbs, onion and seasoning in a coat of pesto sauce!

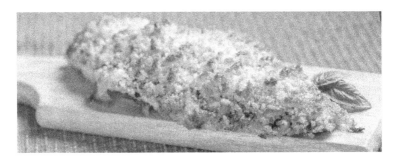

Serving size: 6

Portion: 5

Total time: 20min

Ingredients:

- teaspoons of pesto
- pounds of filleted and boned catfish, 5 to 6oz pieces
- ½ cup of shredded mozzarella cheese
- ¾ cup of panko breadcrumbs
- tablespoons of olive oil

Signature Seasoning Blend of Chef McCargo:

- 1 teaspoon of onion powder
- 1 teaspoon of garlic powder
- ½ teaspoon of red pepper flakes
- ½ teaspoon of dried oregano
- ½ teaspoon of black pepper

Preparation:

Preheat the oven to 400° F.

1. In a small bowl, combine all the seasonings and sprinkle even quantities on both sides of the fish.

2. Spread equivalent quantities of pesto (1 teaspoon) on the top of the fillets and set them aside.

3. Mix the breadcrumbs, cheese and oil in a medium bowl and dredge the pesto side of the fish in the paste until well covered.

4. Liberally grease or coat baking sheet tray with oil and lay side up on foil tray containing fish pesto, leaving some space among filets.

5. Bake on the bottom rack for 15-20 minutes at 400 ° F or until brownness is desired.

6. After cooking, leave to rest for 10 minutes and remove from the tray to avoid breaking the fish.

1.26   3.8 Glazed-Bourbon Skirt Steak

Tired of the same old steak? With Chef McCargo, have your glaze on! To give a mouth-watering taste, mix dark brown sugar, whiskey, butter, Dijon mustard, and spices.

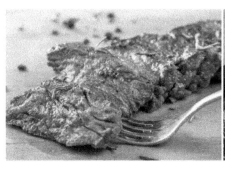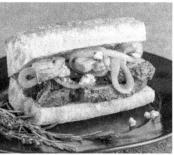

Serving size: 8

Portions: 3

Total time: 20min

Ingredients:

Bourbon Glaze:

- tablespoons of Dijon mustard
- tablespoons of chilled and cubed unsalted butter
- ¼ cup of diced shallots
- ¼ cup of brown sugar
- 1 cup of bourbon
- 1 tablespoon of black pepper

Skirt Steak:

- pounds of skirt steak
- ½ teaspoon of dried oregano
- tablespoons of grape seed oil
- 1 teaspoon of black pepper
- ½ teaspoon of smoked paprika
- 1 tablespoon of red wine vinegar

Preparation:

Bourbon Glaze:

1. On a medium-high flame, brown shallots in 1tsp of butter in a shallow saucepan.

2. Reduce the heat to medium, remove the pan from the burner, add the whiskey, and transfer the sauce to the burner.

3. Cook for 10-15 minutes, or until around one-third part is reduced.

4. Place mustard, brown sugar and black pepper in the mixture and whisk until it becomes bubbly.

5. Turn off the heat and whisk in the remaining 2 teaspoons of cold and cubed butter, stir continuously until well mixed.

Skirt Steak:

1. In a gallon-sized sealable storage container, mix the first 5 ingredients, add steaks, and shake well.

2. Allow the steaks to be marinated in a bag for 30-45 minutes at room temperature.

3. Remove the steaks from the bag, grill each side for 15-20 minutes, then remove and leave for 10 minutes to rest.

Slice and then serve with a sprinkle of sauce or leave whole and brush with some glaze and place in a preheated broiler for 4-6 minutes or until the desired look is achieved

1.27　3.9 Red chili cornbread casserole

To make a taste-bud delight your friends and family won't quickly forget, this casserole mixes fluffy cornbread with spicy chili.

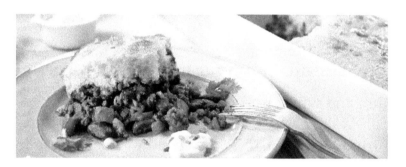

Serving size: 8

Portion: 1

Total time: 15min

Ingredients:

Chili:

- 1 pound of ground beef
- tablespoons of chopped jalapeño peppers
- 1 tablespoon of granulated garlic powder
- ¼ cup of diced celery
- ½ cup of diced onions
- ½ cup of tomato sauce with no added salt

- 1 tablespoon of cumin
- ½ cup of chopped green or red peppers
- 1 tablespoon of chili powder
- tablespoons of dried onion flakes
- 1 cup of shredded cheddar cheese
- 1 teaspoon of ground black pepper
- ¼ cup of water
- 1 cup of rinsed and drained kidney beans
- ¼ cup low-sodium French's Worcestershire sauce

Cornbread:

- ¾ cup of flour
- 1½ tablespoons of unsalted and melted butter
- ¼ cup of cornmeal
- ½ teaspoon of cream of tartar
- ½ cup of sugar
- ¾ cup of milk
- ¼ teaspoon of baking soda
- 1 beaten egg
- ¼ cup of canola oil

Preparation:

1. Brown ground beef in a wide saucepan, with onions, jalapeños celery, and bell peppers. Drain the excess oil. Add the chili powder, flakes, water, garlic powder, cumin, onion, tomato sauce, black pepper, Worcestershire sauce, and beans. For an extra 10 minutes, cook. Remove from the heat and pour into a baking pan measuring 9" x 9" and then layer the cheese.

2. Mix the cornmeal, baking soda, flour, tartar cream and sugar in a medium-sized dish.

3. Put the egg, oil, melted butter, and milk in a small bowl. Fold together the flour mixture and the egg mixture (you might see a few lumps, which is okay, don't overbeat).

4. Pour the mixture over the chili and bake uncovered for 25 minutes, then covered at 350 ° F for 20 minutes and then switch off the oven and allow to rest for 5 minutes.

Chapter no: 4 Renal-friendly chilled fruit salads

Take the lead from your freezer and cool down the summer snacks or meals with a yummy and chilled fruit salad. Since these salads are prepared from fruits low in potassium, they are sufficiently kidney-friendly to serve your next party or daily meals. To prepare these fruity salads, no heat is needed so the kitchen would be cool, and the chef will be smiling!

4.1 Caramel Apple Salad

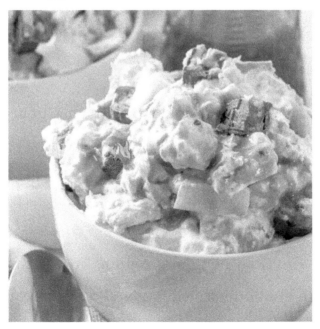

Portions: 10

Diet types include: Lower protein, CKD non-dialysis, Diabetes and Dialysis

Serving Size: 1/2 cup

Totaltime:10min

Ingredients:

- 1/4 cup of butterscotch baking chips
- ounces canned crushed and packed juicy pineapple
- cups of Granny smith apples
- 1/2 cup of butterscotch dessert topping
- ounces of whipped topping
- 1/3 cup of unsalted peanuts

Preparation:

1. Clean the apples, but do not peel them. Cut apples into cubes of around 1'. Thaw the whipped topping.

2. Mix smashed pineapple with diced apples (including juice).

3. Mix the thawed non-dairy topping in a separate large bowl with the butterscotch flavored dessert coating until uniformly spread.

4. In the non-dairy topping combination, stir the apple/pineapple mixture.

5. To the mixture, add unsalted peanuts and butterscotch chips

6. Mix and serve.

Helpful hints:

- Around 2 medium apples produce 3 cups.
- Make it ahead and refrigerate but leave the peanuts out until ready to serve and eat.
- Peanuts are obligatory. If used, ensure that unsalted peanuts are used; salted peanuts can influence the salad's consistency. 32 mg of potassium and 17 mg of phosphorus per serving are provided by 1/3 cup of peanuts.

1.28   4.2 Shrimp noodle and chilled veggie salad

This recipe is so easy and quick to make. Toss together spaghetti and shrimp, shitake, mushrooms, spinach, onions, garlic and fresh ginger. It is a great summer· all-in-one recipe that you can eat for lunch and dinner.

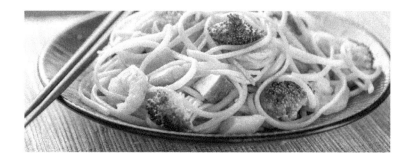

Serving size: 10

Portion: 1 3/4 cup

Total time: 10min

Ingredients:

- 14-ounce pack of cooked salad shrimp or 4 cups of cooked, peeled, tailless and deveined cocktail shrimp and cut in half
- cups of fresh broccoli florets
- 1 cup of sliced on the bias fresh scallions
- cups of chopped fresh shitake mushrooms
- 1 cup of shredded fresh carrots
- teaspoons of chili oil
- 1 pound of package of dry Spaghetti noodles, cooked and chilled but don't rinse
- ½ cup of rice wine vinegar
- 1 tablespoon of chopped fresh ginger

- tablespoons of chopped fresh garlic
- ¼ cup of reduced-sodium soy sauce substitute (recipe below)
- ¼ cup of fresh lime juice (max 2 limes) and zest of 1 lime (1tbsp)
- 2 tablespoons of sesame oil

Low-Sodium Soy Sauce Substitute (makes 1 cup):

- 1 teaspoon of low-sodium soy sauce
- ¼ teaspoon of garlic powder
- teaspoons of Better Than Bouillon low-sodium Chicken Base
- teaspoons of dark molasses
- 1½ cups of water
- ¼ teaspoon of white pepper
- teaspoons of balsamic vinegar
- ¼ teaspoon of ground ginger

Preparation:

1. Combine the substitute soy sauce components in a small saucepan.

2. On medium flame, stir it. Allow it to reduce and slightly thicken to around 1 cup. Store the rest in the freezer.

3. Then, in a large bowl, combine the first six ingredients and set them aside.

4. Blend the rest of the ingredients in the blender until well mixed, around 1 minute.

5. Pour the pasta mixture over the dressing mixture. Toss until it's coated well, then serve.

1.29   4.3 Crunchy and sweet coleslaw

In this fresh twist on traditional coleslaw, celery seed sweet onion, and a splash of mustard, bring spice and crunch. Serve for lunch and dinner

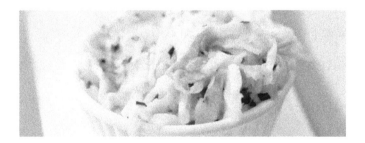

Serving size: 12

Portion: 1

Total time: 10min

Ingredients:

- ½ cup of chopped sweet onion
- cups of shredded cabbage
- 1 cup of canola oil
- ½ cup of rice vinegar
- 1 cup of sugar
- 1 teaspoon of celery seed
- 1 teaspoon of yellow prepared mustard

Preparation:

1. Mix the shredded cabbage in a large bowl with the sliced onion.

2. Blend the other ingredients in a blender until well mixed.

3. Pour the dressing over the cabbage and onion. Mix and refrigerate properly.

4. Only serve it cold.

1.30   4.4 Chicken Fruit Salad

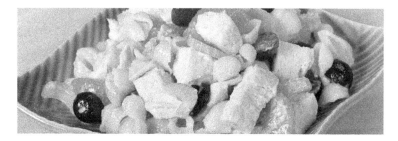

Portions: 8

Diet types include: Diabetes, CKD non-dialysis, Lower protein and dialysis

Serving size: 1-1/3 cups

Total time: 10min

Ingredients:

- 3/4 cup of mayonnaise
- cups of cooked chicken
- ounces of small uncooked shell pasta
- 1-1/2 cups of seedless grapes
- 1-1/2 cups of celery
- 15 ounces of canned mandarin oranges

Preparation:

1. Cube the cooked chicken. Slice the celery into halves and slice the grapes. Drain the oranges mandarin.

2. Pasta is prepared according to the packet, omitting salt. In cold water, rinse and drain to cool. Drain thoroughly.

3. Combine the cooked pasta and all the ingredients in a large bowl. To mix, combine properly.

4. Cover and cool it down before serving.

Chapter no 5: Renal-friendly snack ideas

Snacky feeling? Each of these quick snack selections is kidney-friendly, and they also taste amazing! You will enjoy guilt-free snacks if you consume in balance and make healthy decisions consistent with the kidney health requirements. With your doctor or nutritionist's support, discover what snack foods are healthy for your kidney diet. We all love snacks, of course, don't we? Yet, we recognize that most snacks are also packed with trans (or bad) fat, sugar, calories, salt, and other kidney-harming additives. So, there are some on-the-go finest kidney-friendly snacks listed below. Fortunately, in our fridge and pantry, these foods items are typical things we often have.

1.31   5.1 Cinnamon and orange Biscotti

Enjoy the orange, tangy taste, warmed with a hint of cinnamon and served in a crispy biscotti. Dip in coffee or tea or enjoy it as a dessert or snack.

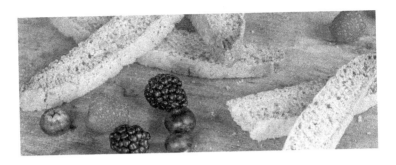

Serving size: 18 cookies

Portion: 1

Total time: 15min

Ingredients:

- 1 cup of sugar
- 2 large eggs
- ½ cup of unsalted butter at room temperature
- 1 teaspoon of vanilla extract
- 2 teaspoons of grated orange peel
- 2 cups of all-purpose flour
- ½ teaspoon of baking soda
- 1 teaspoon of cream of tartar
- ¼ teaspoon of salt
- 1 teaspoon of ground cinnamon

Preparation:

1. Preheat the oven to 325° F.

2. 1.Spray the nonstick cooking spray on 2 baking sheets.

3. In a large bowl, beat the unsalted butter and sugar until well combined.

4. Put eggs one by one, beating it well after each.

5. Whisk together the orange peel and vanilla.

6. In a medium-size dish, combine the flour, tartar cream, cinnamon, baking soda and salt.

7. To the butter mixture, add the dry ingredients and combine until mixed.

8. Cut the dough in two. Place each half on a sheet that has been prepared. Shape each half into a log form that is 3 inches wide and three-quarters of an inch long with lightly floured hands. Bake for around 35 minutes until the dough logs are soft to the touch.

9. Remove the dough logs from the oven and cool for 10 minutes.

10. Move logs to the surface. Cut diagonally into 1/2-inch-thick slices with the help of serrated blades. On baking sheets, place cut side down.

11. Bake for about 12 minutes until the bottoms are golden.

12. Turn over the biscotti; bake for around 12 minutes more until the bottoms are golden.

13. Before serving, transfer it to a wire rack and let it cool.

1.32   5.2 Homemade Herbed Biscuits

Craving some kidney-friendly cookies? There is a recipe. Herbs, some milk and flour, lots of healthy goodness are everything you need for these fluffy and savory biscuits.

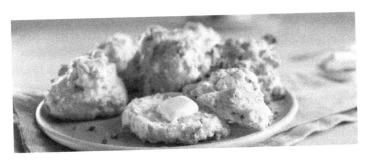

Serving size: 12

Portion: 1

Total time: 20min

Ingredients:

- 1 teaspoon of cream of tartar

- Some nonstick cooking sprays
- 1¾ cups of all-purpose flour
- ¼ cup of mayonnaise
- ⅔ cup of skim milk
- ½ teaspoon of baking soda
- tablespoons of chives or some other herb, dry and fresh to taste

Preparation:

1 Preheat the oven to 400° F. Next, brush the nonstick cooking spray on the baking sheet.

2 Combine the rice, tartar cream and baking soda in a large bowl. Then blend with a fork in the mayonnaise, so the paste appears like coarse cornmeal.

3 Combine the milk and herbs in a small bowl and add them to the flour mixture. Until mixed, stir.

4 Place on the cookie sheet some heaping tablespoons. For 10 minutes, bake them.

5 Until ready to use, refrigerate them.

1.33   5.3 Heavenly Deviled Eggs

This traditional and easy deviled eggs recipe seems to be the way to go if you're searching for a fast and tasty appetizer that is often a crowd-pleaser. Perfect at every moment.

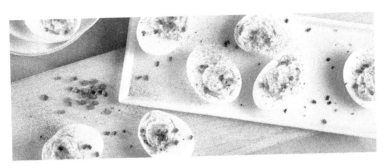

Serving size: 4

Portion: 2

Total time: 15min

Ingredients:

- Dash of paprika for optional garnishing
- tablespoons of light mayonnaise
- large hard-boiled eggs, shells removed
- ¼ teaspoon of ground black pepper
- ½ teaspoon of cider vinegar
- ½ teaspoon of dry mustard
- 1 tablespoon of finely chopped onion

Preparation:

1 Slice the eggs lengthwise in two. Pick the yolks carefully and put them in a small dish. Position the white egg on a tray.

2 Mash the yolks with a fork's help and add the dried vinegar, mustard, onion and black pepper to the yolks.

3 Refill the cooked eggs with the mixture of yolk, heaping gently.

4 Sprinkle paprika on deviled eggs (optional) and then serve.

5.4   Sweet Popcorn Balls

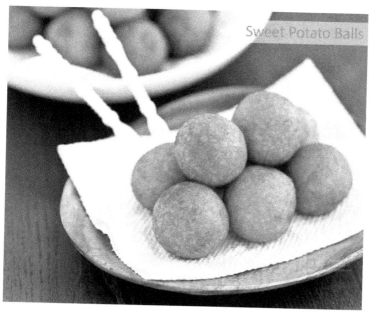

Portions: 18

Serving size: 1 ball of popcorn

Diet type includes: Dialysis, Lower protein, Vegetarian and CKD non-dialysis

Total time: 20min

Ingredients:

- tablespoons of whipped butter
- cups of Karo dark corn syrup
- 16 cups of unsalted popped popcorn
- 1 cup of water
- cups of brown sugar
- 1 tablespoon of vinegar

Preparation:

1 Pop the popcorn and drop it in a wide bowl. Put it aside to use later.

2 In a saucepan, mix the honey, brown sugar, water and vinegar.

3 Cook over medium heat and whisk until the mixture boils while stirring continuously. Continue to cook and mix continuously over medium heat for 15-20 minutes.

4   Cook to the hard stage of a ball (until a small amount of mixture forms hardball when tested in very cold water.)

5   Remove from the oven, add butter quickly, and then stir.

6   Slowly pour the mixture in a large bowl over the popped popcorn while mixing properly. Using as little pressure as possible, shape it into balls.

7   Every popcorn ball is covered in plastic wrap and placed in an airtight jar.

Helpful hints:

Butter hands, and better still, put buttered latex gloves over them. Popcorn is not going to stick as badly, and it's not as hot!

1.34   5.5 Shrimp Spread with Crackers

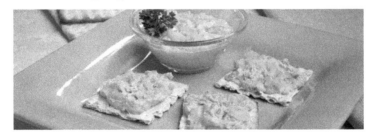

Serving size: Maximum 3 crackers, each with almost 1 teaspoons of spread

Portions: 8

Diet types include: Lower Protein, CKD non-dialysis, Dialysis and A Heart Healthy

Total time: 20min

Ingredients:

- 1/2 teaspoon of Mrs. Dash herb seasoning blend
- 1 tablespoon of parsley
- 1/4 cup of light cream cheese
- 1/4 teaspoon of Tabasco hot sauce
- 1 tablespoon of no-salt-added ketchup
- 1 teaspoon of Worcestershire sauce
- 2-1/2 oz cooked shelled shrimp
- 24 matzo of cracker miniatures

Preparation:

6 Set out the cream cheese to soften it.

7 Mince the shrimp and then stir it into cream cheese

8 Stir in ketchup, Worcestershire sauce, Tabasco sauce, and Mrs. Dash spice seasoning for

9 On each cracker, spread 1 teaspoon of spread. Garnish it with minced parsley.

Chapter no: 6 Renal-friendly desserts

Many civil society organizations and health organizations work together to increase and encourage awareness of kidney disorders and kidney-healthy habits. This initiative responds to the increasing rates in the United States and across the globe with Chronic Kidney Disease. Here are some delicious Renal-friendly desserts for you to enjoy whether you have kidney diseases, renal friendly desserts are here to help.

1.35   6.1 Blueberry Corn Cobbler

It will help make sure you are active and linked to nature by collecting your blueberries. one can stay encouraged to communicate by being mindful of breathing and having time with nature.

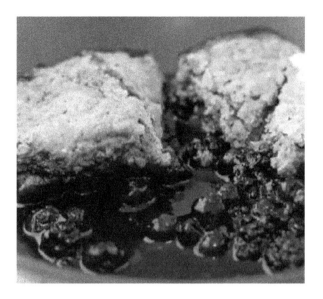

Serving size: 9

Portion: 1 9th of 9-inch square pan

Total time: 20 min

Ingredients:

- 1 egg
- 3/4 cup (170 ml) of honey
- 1/3 cup (79 ml) of milk
- 1/2 tsp of (2.5 g) cream of tartar
- tbsp of (30 g) unsalted butter
- 1 1/4 cup (156 g) of white corn flour
- cups (806 g) of blueberries

- 1/4 tsp of (1.25 g) baking soda

Preparation:

1 Preheat the oven to almost 375 degrees

2 In a mixing bowl, beat up milk, egg, butter, tartar cream, and baking soda.

3 To break up any lumps, add 1/2 cup of the honey and the corn flour while stirring well.

4 In a 9-inch baking dish, spread the berries on the bottom.

5 Drizzle the berries with some of the remaining honey.

6 Drop a tablespoon of batter over the berries.

7 Bake for about 30 to 35 minutes until the crust is lightly browned and the berries have been bubbling.

1.36   6.2 Sweet Crustless Quiche

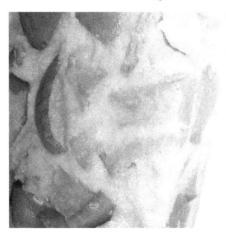

Serving size: 6

Portion: 1/6th of the pie

Total time: 20min

Ingredients:

Basic Crustless Quiche:

- 1 cup of 2% milk (250 ml)
- large eggs
- 1/2 cup of flour (125 g)

Sweet filling:

- 2tbsp of brown sugar
- 1/4 cup of butter
- sliced or diced medium apples

Preparation:

1 In a cup, smash the eggs and whisk in each ingredient, milk, then flour until maximum lumps are smoothed out.
2 If required, add salt, pepper and spices.
3 **Note:** This mixture could be baked and served on its own.

4   On moderate flame, cook the filling ingredients in a skillet until heated and bubbling for around 15-20 minutes.

5   A deep-dish pie tray or an 8-8-inch baking pan with cooking spray is heavily covered, so sure it is properly coated or else the quiche can stick.

6   Pour into the greased baking pan the cooked filing (2-3 cups) and scatter thinly to distribute uniformly.

7   Cover with the mixture of crustless quiche and bake for 40-45 minutes at 350 degrees until a knife comes out dry and the top is golden brown.

1.37   6.3 Apple and Blueberry Crisp

A perfect way to enjoy summer is to get crisps and crumbles. Bring this meal to a barbecue or picnic and make new friends for sure.

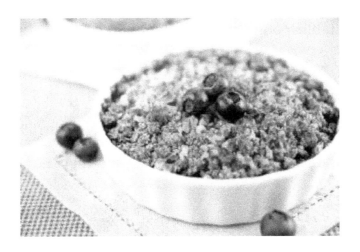

Serving size: 8

Portion: 1/4 cup of crumble and 1/2 cup of cooked fruit

Total time: 20min

Ingredients:

Crisp:

- 1/4 cup or (60 ml) brown sugar
- 1 1/4 cups or (310 ml) quick cooking rolled oats
- tablespoons or (90 ml) non-hydrogenated melted margarine
- 1/4 cup or (60 ml) all-purpose flour (unbleached)

Filling:

- teaspoons or (20 ml) cornstarch

- 1 tablespoon or (15 ml) lemon juice

- 1/2 cup or (125 ml) brown sugar

- cups or (500 ml) chopped or grated apples

- cups frozen or fresh non-thawed blueberries

- 1 tablespoon or (15 ml) melted margarine

Preparation:

1. Preheat the oven to 350 °F with the rack in the center position.

2. Combine the dried products in a bowl. Add the butter and whisk until the mixture is just moistened, then put it aside.

3. Mix the brown sugar and cornstarch in a 20-cm (8-inch) square baking dish.

4. Add the lemon juice and berries and toss to blend.

5. Apply the crisp mixture to the surface and bake for about 55 minutes to 1 hour or until golden brown.

6. Serve cold or warm.

1.38   6.4 Berry Oatmeal Muffins

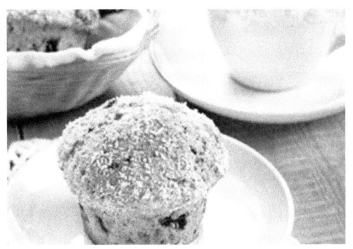

Serving size: 12

Portion: 1 muffin

Total time: 20min

Ingredients:

- 125 ml or (1/2 cup) quick-cooking oatmeal
- 250 ml or (1 cup) all-purpose flour (unbleached)
- 2.5 ml or (1/2 tsp) baking soda
- 160 ml or (2/3 cup) lightly packed brown sugar
- 125 ml or (1/2 cup) applesauce
- 2 eggs
- 60 ml or (1/4 cup) canola oil
- 1 lemon with the grated zest

- 1 orange (grated zest only)
- 180 ml or (3/4 cup) of frozen or fresh raspberries
- 180 ml or (3/4 cup) of frozen or fresh blueberries
- 15 ml or (1 tbsp) of lemon juice

Preparation:

1. Preheat the oven to 180°C (350°F) with the rack in the central spot. Line about 12 muffin cups with liners of paper or silicone.
2. Mix the rice, brown sugar, oatmeal and baking soda in a dish. Set it aside.
3. Eggs, oil, applesauce, lemon juice and citrus zest are whisked in a large bowl. Stir the dry ingredients using a wooden spoon. Add the berries and softly mix.
4. Scoop in the muffin cups. Bake for about 20 to 22 minutes or until a toothpick placed in the middle of the muffin comes out dry. Enable it to cool.
5. Note* Users also noticed that using a regular-sized muffin baking pan, the more approximate output of this recipe is approx. 6 muffins. Taking this into

account, based on the real yield outcomes, the nutritional values can be improved.

1.39 6.5 Raspberry Cheesecake Mousse

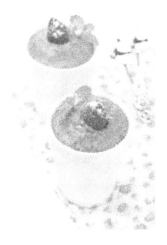

Serving size: 6

Portion: 107 g

Total time 20min

Ingredients:

- 1 cup frozen or fresh raspberries
- 1 8oz pkg. cream cheese kept at room temperature
- 1 cup of light, whipped topping
- 1 tsp of lemon zest finely grated

- 3⁄4 cup of SPLENDA Granular, No Calorie Sweetener
- 1 tsp of vanilla extract

Preparation:

1. Beat the cream cheese until soft and beat until molten in 1/2 cup of the SPLENDA® Granular. Mix the lemon zest and vanilla.

2. For garnish, reserve some raspberries. With a fork, crush the remaining raspberries and stir in the remaining 1⁄4 cup of SPLENDA® Granular until melt.

3. Fold lightly, whipped topping in the cream cheese mixture and fold in the crushed raspberries gently but quickly.

4. In six serving glasses, spoon the mousse and cool before ready to eat.

5. Before eating, garnish the mousse with a sprig of fresh mint and fresh raspberries

1.40   6.6 Almond Meringue Cookies

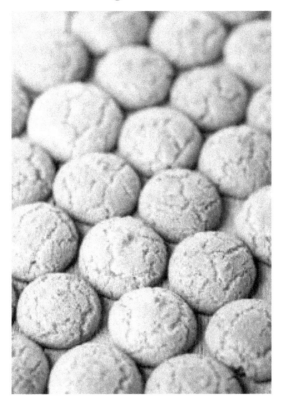

Here is a recipe for Cookies with Almond Meringue to make you fulfill your craving for nuts without all the nuts! Flavor extracts are a perfect way to get the flavor without potassium or phosphorus, such as maple extract or almond extract.

Serving size: 24 small cookies

Portion: 2 small cookies

Total time: 20min

Ingredients:

- tbsp of pasteurized egg whites or 2 egg whites (allow them to come to room temperature)
- ½ tsp of almond extract
- 1 tsp of cream of tartar
- ½ cup of white sugar
- ½ tsp of vanilla extract

Preparation:

1. Preheat the oven to 300F.
2. Beat the egg whites with tartar cream until the volume has doubled. Add the rest of the ingredients and beat till they form firm peaks.
3. using two teaspoons, Push a teaspoon full of meringue with the back of another spoon onto a parchment-lined baking sheet.
4. Bake for around 25 minutes at 300F or until the meringues are crisp. Store in an airtight jar.

1.41   6.7 Molten Mint Chocolate Brownies

This super brownie recipe begins with a blend, but it contains a minty, melted chocolate surprise in the middle. It melt-in-your-mouth awesomely.

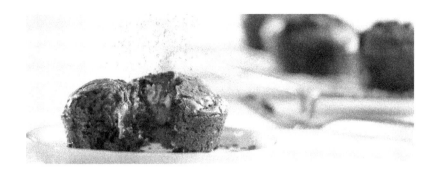

Serving size: 12

Portion: 1.5oz

Total time: 20min

Ingredients:

- 12 Andes mint chocolate
- 1 box of Non-supreme Betty Crocker brownie mix
- Powdered sugar, fresh mint sprigs and cocoa powder (sweetened or unsweetened) as an optional garnish

Preparation:

1   Preheat the oven and cook the brownie mix according to the box's instructions.

2 Prepare a lining or finely greased 12 cup muffin pan and flour the bottom and sides. Into the bowls, pour the brownie mix and bake for 25 minutes.

3 Place one slice of mint candy in the middle and bake for an extra 5 minutes. Remove the brownies from the oven. Switch the oven off and take it out. For 5–10 minutes, let it cool.

4 Take the brownie cupcakes out of the pan, then serve.

5 Optional: Dust some chocolate powder and powdered sugar and garnish with fresh mint and dust.

1.42   6.8 Festive Cream Cheese Sugar Cookies

Make these plain, classic, and enjoyable sugar cookies, and it will seem like a holiday every day. Use cookie cutters, playful and simple, then sprinkle some colored sugar.

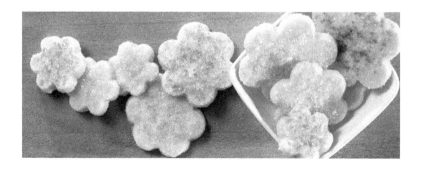

Serving size: 48

Portion: 1

Total time: 20min

Ingredients:

- 1 cup of sugar
- 1 large egg
- 3 ounces of softened cream cheese
- ¼ teaspoon of almond extract
- ½ teaspoon of salt
- 2¼ cups of all-purpose flour
- ½ teaspoon of vanilla extract
- 1 cup of softened and unsalted butter
- Colored sugar for optional garnishing

Preparation:

1. Place the butter, sugar, cream cheese, almond extract, salt, vanilla extract, and egg yolk in a large bowl. Blend thoroughly. Stir in the flour until it is well-mixed.

2. Chill the cookie dough in the fridge for 2 hours.

3. Preheat the oven to 350° F.

4. Roll out the pastry, one-third at a time to 1/4-inch width, on a thinly floured surface. Break using thinly floured cookie cutters into desired shapes.

5. Put them on ungreased cookie sheets 1 inch apart. Brush with gently beaten egg white and sprinkle some colored sugar, keeping cookies plain.

6. For 7–9 minutes or till light golden brown, bake cream cheese cookies. Before serving, let cool totally

Conclusion

The constant struggle to achieve benefits is one of the main causes that impact patients' health rather than care. So, here's a diet that not only lowers health hazards but also keeps an individual healthier. Following a kidney diet tends to support the kidney's functioning and slow the progression of full kidney failure, so the renal diet is best suited. One that is poor in salt, potassium, and protein is a renal diet best for some kidney diseases. A renal diet often stresses the value of eating high-quality protein and typically limiting liquid. The nutritional nature of ketoacid supplementation and renal diet combined with dietary manipulation, including phosphorus, protein and sodium restriction, can exert a cardiovascular protective impact in patients with chronic renal disease by acting on conventional and non-traditional cardiovascular risk factors. The regulation of blood pressure can be favored by decreasing the dietary consumption of sodium, potassium and phosphorus, which is therefore very important for reducing serum cholesterol and improving the lipid profile of plasma. Low consumption of protein and phosphorus has a key function to play in decreasing proteinuria and avoiding and overcoming hyperphosphatemia and secondary hyperparathyroidism, which have been the primary causes of vascular calcification, heart injury and risk of uremic mortality. Therefore, leaving aside the already debatable impact on renal disease development, adequate dietary care or a kidney-friendly diet i-e, Renal diet early during renal disease, can be effective in lowering the incidence of cardiovascular in patients with renal disease. Ultimately, the safest diet for kidney diseases and other health issues is the one that a person practices to reach and sustain a healthy lifestyle, so the Renal diet is a strong and productive way to cope with severe kidney diseases like CKD and stay healthy at the end of the day. You are not going to be disappointed.

CPSIA information can be obtained
at www.ICGtesting.com
Printed in the USA
BVHW040608100321
602119BV00005B/848

9 781801 842150